KETO SEAFOOD

AND FISH RECIPES

Discover the Secrets to Incredible Low-Carb

Fish and Seafood Recipes for Your Keto

Lifestyle

By: Amy Moore

Table of Contents

Introduction:
Enjoying Fish and Seafood on the Keto Diet

The keto diet is a low-carb, high-fat diet that allows you to eat different kinds of foods—but also requires you to avoid certain types of foods, particularly those high in carbs. Basically, your diet would consist mainly of fats, moderate amounts of protein, and minimal amounts of carbs—only enough to survive without becoming nutrient deficient.

If you follow the keto diet, you may have found yourself struggling at one point or another. This is especially true when you can't find enough variety and you start feeling bored with eating the same things over and over again. Then, you start thinking about the foods you used to eat, and you feel a strong urge to give in to your cravings.

If this situation sounds familiar, don't worry—you're not alone. A lot of first-time keto followers have felt this way at some point or another. But the good news is that you don't have to give up your diet. This book is here to help you out. One of the most effective ways to motivate yourself is by making your diet more interesting. Do this by finding different kinds of keto-friendly foods, dishes, and recipes to give yourself the variety you need to stick with your new lifestyle.

Purchasing this book is an excellent move towards improving your health and reaching ketosis, so congratulations! In this book, you'll learn everything you need to know about eating fish and seafood on the keto diet. Fish and seafood are excellent protein sources, they contain good amounts of fat, and they also contain other important nutrients to make you healthy and strong.

In the first chapter, we focus on fish. We start by introducing you to the best types of fish to consume on the keto diet—and the ones you should avoid. This chapter also contains information about the benefits of consuming fish on the keto diet. The second chapter is similar to the first—but this time, we focus on other types of seafood. As you will soon learn, most types of fish and seafood are recommended on the keto diet. These food groups generally contain low amounts of carbs, which is why they are perfect for the ketogenic diet. After these short but highly informative chapters, we get to the good stuff—the main reason why you've chosen to purchase this book in the first place.

In the third chapter, you will learn several keto-friendly dishes featuring different types of fish as their main ingredient. There are recipes featuring salmon, mahi-mahi, tuna, sardines, halibut, tilapia, cod, sea bass, swordfish, and other types of white fish. The great thing about these recipes is that you can substitute the main fish ingredient with similar types of fish based on your own preferences. These recipes are healthy, easy to make, require simple ingredients, and are all bursting with flavors. If you're a fan of fish, learning how to make these scrumptious dishes will enrich your diet and make it a lot easier to follow.

In the next chapter, you will continue your learning process—this time, by learning how to create several seafood dishes. There are recipes that feature scallops, lobster, shrimps, crabs, clams, oysters, and even a recipe where you can combine fish and seafood in a hearty, healthy dish. Just reading these recipes will make your mouth water —and might even make you run to the grocery store to buy all the ingredients you need to make them.

Short as this book is, it contains a wealth of information to help add variety to your ketogenic diet. Any of these dishes will make you feel happy with your decision to go keto. Another benefit you can get from this book is that it contains simple recipes that will help hone your cooking skills. After practicing those skills with these easy recipes, you can level-up your cooking game by finding more complicated ones.

Soon, you'll come to realize that the keto diet isn't difficult at all. In fact, you might even start wondering why you didn't make cooking part of your lifestyle sooner! Cooking can be an enjoyable and fulfilling experience. When you cook your own food, you can be sure that you are only consuming foods that are suitable for your diet. With that being said, let's begin!

Chapter 1:

What Kinds of Fish Can You Eat on Keto?

What is one important thing that salmon, tuna, halibut, and other fish have that makes them ideal for the ketogenic lifestyle? They're an excellent source of vitamins, high-quality proteins, essential fatty acids, and are considered healthy foods. These fish and more also serve as an excellent main ingredient for creating healthy and tasty keto-friendly dishes. Fish is delicious, versatile, and fits right in to your new diet.

When it comes to protein sources, fish is one of the healthiest types of food to include in your diet. The protein you can get from fish is high-quality, and also contains other essential nutrients. And if you opt for fattier types of fish, you would also be consuming high amounts of vitamin D and omega-3. Although cooking fish dishes may seem complicated, you will soon discover that this doesn't always have to be the case.

Later, we will be going through some simple dishes that feature different kinds of healthy and tasty fish. Fish is an excellent food choice because you can do virtually anything with it—bake it, grill it, boil it, broil it, fry it, and more. No matter how you choose to cook your fish, you're sure to end up with a tasty dish for yourself and your whole family.

Types of Fish to Eat

If you want to stay healthy, it's recommended to eat fish at least two times a week. Fish is a healthy and lean protein source that also contains healthy oils and other important nutrients. When it comes to eating fish on the ketogenic diet, there are many options for you. Since most fish are low-carb, you don't have to worry about ruining your diet by eating more fish. Here are some of the best types of fish to consume:

1. Albacore Tuna (especially from British Columbia or the US)

Most types of tuna may contain high levels of mercury, except for this type. When purchasing albacore tuna, go for those which have been pole- or troll-caught to make sure they contain lower levels of mercury and other contaminants.

2. Mackerel

This is a fatty type of fish that would fit perfectly into your diet. In terms of mercury content, Atlantic mackerel contains lower levels compared to Spanish and King mackerel. Therefore, it's recommended to go for this variety. Mackerel is cheaper than salmon, so you may use this as a substitute for some salmon recipes.

3. Rainbow Trout (farmed)

Unfortunately, lake trout contain high levels of contaminants, therefore, it's better to look for farmed rainbow trout. Fortunately, this is the type of trout you will commonly find in fish markets.

4. Salmon (Alaska wild-caught or US freshwater Coho)

Wild-caught salmon from Alaska is healthier and more sustainable than any other kind of salmon being sold in markets. If you can't find this, the next best thing is US freshwater Coho Salmon. This fish is very popular—and for good reason. Salmon contains high amounts of healthy fats, making it perfect for the ketogenic diet. It's also tasty—whether cooked or raw—and you can use it in a wide range of dishes.

5. Sardines (wild-caught from the Pacific)

This tiny and inexpensive fish is becoming more and more popular as it makes its way into several lists of "superfoods." Small as this fish is, it contains more omega-3s per serving than tuna or salmon. It's also one of the very few types of food that naturally contains high levels of vitamin D. Sardines can also be used in different recipes—you can even eat them straight from the can!

Apart from these healthy fish, there are other types of fish you can eat on the ketogenic diet in moderate amounts. The main reason for this is that these fish don't contain as many fats as the ones we have already discussed. But if you use them with dishes that include butter, olive oil, and other healthy fats, then you may choose to eat them more frequently. These fish include:

1. Catfish

Catfish is a lean type of fish that contains a good amount of protein. It's a low-calorie fish that you may enjoy occasionally while on keto. However, you may have to make up for its low fat content by having it with a high-fat side dish. Also, consider the protein content of this fish as you count your macros for the day.

2. Cod

Cod is another lean type of fish that contains more protein than fat. You may consume cod to hit your protein recommendation for the day, but it's not recommended for when you still have to consume a lot of fats to complete your daily requirement. However, it does go well with fatty ingredients like butter and oil. So if you want to increase the fat content of your meal, make sure to cook dishes that incorporate these healthy fats, too.

3. Tilapia

This is another type of fish that packs a good protein punch. While low in fat, tilapia is tasty, versatile, and easy to cook. If you need to limit your caloric intake for the day, this fish is an excellent choice. But as with the other types of low-fat fish, you should use high-fat ingredients when cooking tilapia to make it more keto-friendly.

Here are other types of fish you may consume moderately while on keto. Again, if you want to make them more suitable for your diet, cook them with high-fat ingredients!

- Anchovies

- Eel

- Flounder

- Haddock

- Halibut

- Herring

- Mahi-mahi

- Perch

- Pollock

- Red Snapper

- Rockfish

- Sea bass

- Skate

- Sole

- Tilefish

- Turbot

Types of Fish to Limit or Avoid

While most types of fish are recommended on the ketogenic diet, there are some you may want to limit or avoid. The reason for this recommendation isn't because they aren't suitable for the diet. Instead, it's recommended to avoid these fish because they either contain high PCB and mercury levels, or their populations are being rapidly depleted. These fish are:

1. Bluefin Tuna

In 2009, this particular tuna species was placed on the WWF's list of threatened wildlife species. Bluefin tuna also contains high levels of PCBs and mercury, making it unsuitable for consumption.

2. Grouper

This is another type of fish that contains high mercury levels. Also, groupers don't reproduce as frequently as other types of fish, which makes them at risk for overfishing.

3. Monkfish

This is a strange-looking fish that dwells at the bottom of the sea. Unfortunately, it has a fresh and light taste, making it a popular fish for gourmet dishes. But, like bluefin tuna, this species of fish is in danger of being depleted, which is why it's recommended to limit or avoid consumption.

4. Orange Roughy

Like grouper, this type of fish reproduces slowly, thus placing it at risk for overfishing. Orange roughy also contains high mercury levels, so you shouldn't be eating a lot of this fish, anyway.

5. Patagonian Toothfish or Chilean Sea Bass

This is a very popular type of fish to eat because it has buttery meat. Unfortunately, the methods by which Patagonian toothfish are caught damages the ocean floors and causes harm to seabirds. Also, it contains high levels of mercury.

6. Salmon (farmed)

Although wild-caught salmon is recommended for its health benefits, farmed salmon isn't. This type of salmon has high PCB levels and are given antibiotics during the farming process.

Benefits of Eating Fish

Adding fish to your ketogenic diet enriches it and makes it healthier. Most types of fish are low in carbs, contain good amounts of protein, and some of them are even high in fats. Aside from this, fish also contains other healthy nutrients the body needs to function well. Here are the benefits of eating fish:

1. There is a wide range of options to choose from

When it comes to fish, there are so many different types available that can be incorporated into your diet. And you can use these different types of fish in different dishes—and cook them in different ways. Also, you don't have to worry about breaking the bank when buying fish. Fresh fish is relatively affordable— unless you opt for the rare or expensive types of fish.

Generally, though, you can purchase fresh, frozen, canned, or bottled fish from different stores to use for your fish recipes. If you live in an area near the seaside, then you have access to a wider range of options. Visit your local shops and see what's available. The great thing about fish is that you can substitute them in recipes as long as you choose fish with a similar taste or texture as the one required in the recipe.

2. Fish is rich in omega-3 and other fatty acids

Most fish contains high levels of omega-3 fatty acids and other types of fatty acids, too (depending on the fish). This is an excellent benefit because these fatty acids have a significant positive impact on your overall health—especially on your heart health. Omega fatty acids can help reduce your risk of stroke and heart disease, lower the levels of triglycerides and blood pressure, and raise the levels of beneficial HDL cholesterol.

Getting enough omega-3 fatty acids each day also has a positive effect on your mental health. This beneficial fatty acid can help combat anxiety, depression, and can even help manage the symptoms of ADHD in children. Omega-3s can lower the risk of developing Alzheimer's disease and other types of brain diseases, as well. Another good effect is that omega-3s can help lower inflammation and the risk of developing various autoimmune diseases.

When it comes to omega-3s and other types of fatty acids, the most beneficial types of fish are the fattier types. Apart from providing these fatty acids, fatty types of fish also fit in perfectly with your ketogenic diet. Since these fish also contain protein, you can keep eating fatty fish to enjoy this particular benefit and more.

3. Fish contains other essential micronutrients, too

The specific amounts of micronutrients of fish depends on the type you have chosen to cook and consume. Generally, though, most fish contains essential vitamins, minerals, and nutrients. This is why fish is considered a superfood, too. Different types of fish contain iodine, selenium, vitamin D, vitamin A, B-vitamins, zinc, iron, and more. For smaller fish, you don't have to remove the bones to eat them—this means that you're getting calcium, as well. Calcium is important for the health of the teeth and bones. But it's also important for the rhythm of your heart, proper blood clotting, and muscle function.

4. Fish contains good amounts of protein

Finally, fish contains good amounts of protein, too—especially the low-fat fish varieties. This helps preserve your lean body mass while maintaining the proper functioning of your organs and tissues. If you have already consumed enough fats for the day, your final meal can be a dish with a lean type of fish to up your protein intake.

Tips for Buying Fresh Fish

When it comes to buying fish for cooking, you must make sure to purchase the freshest fish available. This is important, especially for meal planning so you can store the dishes you have cooked for a longer time. Also, fresh fish just tastes better! Typically, whole fish are the freshest and the most affordable. Therefore, you may want to purchase one whole fish then have it filleted, rather than buying pre-cut fish. Here are some things to look out for when checking for freshness:

- Check out the catch of the day or ask the seller which fish is the freshest.

- Look for shiny and firm flesh—when you touch the flesh, it should bounce back.

- Give the fish a sniff—it shouldn't have a "fishy" smell, but a fresh, ocean-breeze smell.

- The eyes should be clear and bulge a bit.

- The gills should be wet and bright red or pink in color.

- For fish steaks and fillets, they should have a consistent color throughout and should be moist to the touch.

- Also, the flesh shouldn't have gaps or separations for steaks and fillets.

- Whether whole or cut up, the fish shouldn't have a spongy texture, discoloration, and yellow or brown edges.

Once you reach home—and you don't plan to cook your fish yet—use plastic wrap to wrap the fish tightly. Then, set the fish on ice and place it in the refrigerator until it's time to cook.

Chapter 2:
What Kinds of Seafood Can You Eat on Keto?

As with fish, most types of seafood are low in carbs and have sufficient amounts of fat and protein. In fact, there are certain types of seafood that don't contain any carbs—like shrimp and some kinds of crab. While shellfish may contain some carbs, you can still eat them as long as you take note of the number of carbs they contain and include this number into your daily macronutrient count.

When it comes to choosing seafood for your keto diet, make sure it's fresh. That way, you can experience the natural flavors of the seafood without the fishy taste. Also, if you practice meal planning and you start with fresh ingredients, you can store your cooked dishes in the refrigerator for a while without worrying that your prepared meals will spoil. Seafood is another versatile food group, as you can cook seafood in different ways and use this in different dishes.

If you're planning to make fish and seafood a staple part of your keto diet, you may want to visit your local supermarkets, farmer's markets, and seafood stores. That way, you know exactly what types of seafood are readily available in your area—and those which are harder to come by. That way, it's easier for you to plan your meals and know the recipes you can easily whip up for your daily meals, for parties, and for other occasions.

Types of Seafood to Eat

Seafood is an excellent food option for the keto diet. It contains healthy protein, healthy fats, and most types of seafood are low in carbs. Of course, the carb content of seafood varies depending on the type of seafood—the key is to know how many carbs the seafood you plan to use for your recipes contain and add that to your daily total for the day. This is the same thing you would do for other types of food, too, when you're following the ketogenic diet.

The great thing about seafood is that there are so many choices available. When you use seafood as the main protein source of your dishes, you can change up other ingredients and create a new dish just by adding a different seafood choice. While you can consume many different types of seafood on the keto diet, here are some of the best options:

1. Mussels

Even though mussels contain carbs, they are very healthy and make an excellent addition to the ketogenic diet. Mussels contain several essential micronutrients like B-vitamins, manganese, iron, phosphorus, and selenium. Also, despite being low in calories, mussels can be quite filling. So having a mussel dish occasionally can be a great addition to your ketogenic diet—especially if one of your goals is to lose weight.

2. Oysters (farmed)

Farmed oysters are an excellent choice because they are high in iron and omega-3s. They're even beneficial to the environment! Oysters naturally feed off the algae and nutrients in the water, which enhances the water's quality. Oysters even act as natural reefs to attract and provide food for other types of fish. But when it comes to oysters, just make sure that if you eat them raw, you have purchased them from a clean source. That way, you don't have to worry about getting sick because of bacteria.

3. Shrimp

This is the most common type of seafood used in dishes—and it comes in multiple varieties. Although some people find it a hassle to remove the peel of shrimps, the nutritional benefits they offer are definitely worth the effort. Apart from protein and fat, shrimp also contains vitamin D, selenium, B-vitamins, iron, and copper. Even though shrimps contain cholesterol, too, you don't have to be afraid of this fact. Studies have shown that consuming shrimp may lower your triglycerides and may also improve the ratio of HDL to LDL.

Apart from these seafood options, there are other nutrient-dense types of seafood that are high in fat and protein and low in carbs, and so would fit in well with your ketogenic diet. These include:

- Abalone
- Caviar
- Clams
- Crab
- Lobster
- Scallops
- Squid

Types of Seafood to Limit or Avoid

Seafood is one of the healthiest and most nutrient-dense types of food out there. Food that comes from the sea contains vitamins, minerals, and other good stuff, giving them high nutritional value. When it comes to seafood, you may consume any variety while following the ketogenic diet. Opt for those which contain low amounts of carbs and for those which do contain some carbs, you may moderate your consumption. Despite this freedom to consume different types of seafood, there are some risks to consider when it comes to seafood consumption:

1. Allergies

This is one of the most common dangers of eating seafood—having an allergic reaction. If this is your first time eating seafood, you may want to consume a small amount, then observe your body for any adverse allergic reactions. While there's a very small likelihood that you'll be allergic to all types of seafood, you may have such a reaction to some varieties. In such a case, simply avoid the type of seafood you're allergic to so you don't have to suffer through the reaction and all of its symptoms.

2. Methylmercury

The pollution of the environment has caused several varieties of fish and seafood to be contaminated with mercury—a kind of neurotoxin. While this issue is more common in fish than in other kinds of seafood, it's still worth noting. Consuming foods that contain mercury is particularly troubling for pregnant women and developing children. So, if you want to avoid this risk, choose your seafood carefully and always check the sources.

Benefits of Eating Seafood

Just as consuming fish can be very beneficial to your health, consuming seafood can also be very beneficial. According to the American Heart Association, consuming seafood at least two times each week may significantly lower your risk of stroke and heart attack. This applies whether you're following the ketogenic diet or any other kind of diet. This fact isn't surprising at all, since seafood contains a lot of anti-inflammatory and heart-healthy omega-3s compared to most other types of foods. If you're following the ketogenic diet, including seafood into it should be very easy, because most seafood is low-carb. Also, seafood is extremely versatile, so you can use it in many different types of dishes—a few of which you will learn later on.

The term seafood often refers to both saltwater and freshwater shellfish—sometimes, it even includes fish. But plants that grow in the sea, such as seaweed and edible algae, can also be considered seafood. Consuming seafood on the ketogenic diet helps give your omega-3 intake a boost. Omega-3s and other fatty acids are essential to health because your body cannot produce them on its own. Therefore, in order to get these fatty acids, you must consume foods that contain them.

Seafood contains an omega-3 fatty acid known as DHA. This is an important component for the skin, retina, sperm, and brain. Seafood is also a high-quality protein source, as well as an excellent source of important minerals, B-vitamins, antioxidants, and fat-soluble vitamins. Here are the other benefits to look forward to when eating seafood:

1. Improves the health of your brain

As previously mentioned, seafood is an excellent source of DHA. According to research, DHA has a very unique and important role in the neuron membranes of the brain. DHA is also essential for the healthy growth and development of the brain. It can even help protect the brain against aging and the development of neurodegenerative diseases.

2. Helps prevent diseases

There are several diseases—such as obesity, cardiovascular disease, diabetes, and some forms of cancer—that you can prevent by making positive changes to your lifestyle and diet. For instance, eating more seafood and fish can help reduce your risk of developing these conditions and other kinds of health problems. According to researchers, the most preventive benefits of seafood come from its high levels of omega-3 fatty acids.

Plant seafood, such as algae and seaweed, also offer some unique benefits. These contain high levels of phytochemicals and antioxidants. Some of these sea plants are also high in iodine, a nutrient that's essential for the health of the thyroid gland. Seaweed contains omega-3s, as well, but in minimal amounts.

3. Higher vitamin D intake

As with fish, seafood is an excellent source of vitamin D3. This form of vitamin D is the most bioavailable and is essential for metabolic, bone, and immune health. Since vitamin D3 is fat-soluble, it's more commonly found in fish and seafood that are high in fat.

Tips for Buying Fresh Seafood

When it comes to buying seafood—and some types of fish—you have the choice to buy fresh or frozen products. This is especially important if you live in a place that doesn't have ready access to fresh seafood. Also, some recipes may require frozen seafood—all you have to do is thaw the meat as part of the preparation process. Whether you plan to buy fresh or frozen seafood, here are some tips for you:

1. For fresh seafood

   O Fresh clams, mussels, and oysters are typically sold live since their internal organs deteriorate quickly after they die. Therefore, when buying these types of seafood, make sure the shells are closed and unbroken. The shells should be moist, shiny, and have a subtle sweet smell.

   O Oysters which have been freshly shucked must smell fresh and have a light grey liquid surrounding them.

○ In the same way, crabs and lobsters are also sold live, since they tend to spoil quickly after dying. Therefore, you must make sure that this seafood should still be moving upon purchase.

○ For shrimps, they should have a mild smell and firm meat. The shells mustn't have dark areas, blackened edges, or black spots.

○ For squid, choose the ones with full and clear eyes, cream-colored skin with brownish-red spots, and firm flesh.

2. For frozen seafood

○ Frozen seafood should be packed in a moisture-proof, close-fitting package. If the packaging is crushed or torn, don't purchase.

○ When taking frozen seafood from a store's freezer, choose the ones below the load line.

○ Bring a cooler with ice to the supermarket to prevent the defrosting of your seafood as you transport it home. This especially important if you live far away from the store.

Chapter 3:
Keto-Friendly Fish Recipes

Now that you know more about eating fish and other seafood on keto, it's time to learn some tasty, healthy, and easy recipes to enrich your new diet. In this chapter, we will go through various recipes that feature different kinds of fish as their main ingredient. If you love fish and you just can't wait to enjoy the health benefits, you can start whipping up these interesting dishes!

Cucumber Noodles with Thyme-Ghee Baked Salmon

This baked dish is simple, easy to make, and so flavorful. It's full of beneficial and essential fatty acids from the wild salmon that serves as the star of this dish. Salmon is an excellent source of protein, and it's so versatile, too!

Time: 20 minutes

Serving Size: 2 servings

Ingredients:

- 2 tbsp olive oil
- 3 tbsp butter or ghee
- ½ cup green olives (pitted)
- salt
- thyme leaves (fresh)
- 1 large cucumber
- 1 whole fennel bulb (sliced roughly)
- 2 salmon fillets (wild, with skin)

Directions:

1. Preheat your oven to 350°F and line an oven tray with parchment paper.

2. Add the sliced fennel to the oven tray, place the salmon fillets on top, and dot the salmon with butter (or ghee). Then, sprinkle with thyme leaves.

3. Place the tray in the oven and bake the salmon for about 15 minutes.

4. While baking the salmon, use a spiralizer to create cucumber noodles. Gently squeeze the noodles to drain excess liquid.

5. Place the cucumber noodles in a bowl, dress with olive oil, and toss to coat evenly. Transfer the cucumber noodles onto plates.

6. Take the tray out of the oven and place the salmon fillets on top of the noodles. Sprinkle with salt and top with olives.

Beurre Blanc Mahi-Mahi

This keto-friendly entrée will tickle your taste buds with its rich and buttery sauce. Fancy as the name of this dish might sound, it's really easy to make. Whether you plan to cook this for yourself or those you love, this dish will surely impress.

Time: 20 minutes

Serving Size: 6 servings

Ingredients:

- 1 tbsp dill (fresh, chopped)

- 2 tbsp parsley (fresh, chopped)

- ¼ cup heavy cream

- ¼ cup olive oil

- ¼ cup white wine

- 1 lemon (juiced)

- 1 stick of butter (sliced)

- 3 strips of bacon

- 6 mahi-mahi fillets

- salt

- pepper

Directions:

1. Fry the bacon strips for about 5 minutes until crispy. Chop the bacon. Set the bacon and the fat aside separately.

2. Use pepper and salt to season the mahi-mahi fillets. Season generously for best results.

3. In a skillet, heat olive oil on medium-high heat. Once hot, sear the mahi-mahi fillets for 3 minutes on each side.

4. Leave the skillet on the heat, but transfer the fillets to a plate.

5. Add the white wine and reduce to a syrup.

6. Add the bacon fat and heavy cream and turn the heat off. Whisk in the pieces of

butter to melt and incorporate fully into the sauce.

7. Add the herbs, lemon juice, bacon, pepper, and salt, then mix well.

8. Pour the sauce over the cooked mahi-mahi fillets and serve immediately.

Tuna Bowl with Roasted Broccoli and Cauliflower

One of the simplest, easiest, and tastiest ways to prepare vegetables is by roasting them. This softens the veggies so that they can absorb more flavors when cooked. This is exactly what you will do to the veggies in this recipe. Prepare for a filling and flavor-rich dish—with tuna as its star.

Time: 25 minutes

Serving Size: 4 bowls

Ingredients for the tuna bowl:

- ¼ cup parsley (fresh, finely chopped)
- 1 broccoli head (broken into florets)
- 1 cauliflower head (broken into florets)
- 1 lemon
- 4 cans of tuna (5-ounces each, packed in olive oil or brine)
- olive oil
- salt

Ingredients for sauce:

- 1 tbsp sesame oil

- 3 tbsp tamari soy sauce

- ¼ cup tahini

Directions:

1. Preheat your oven to 400°F and line a baking tray with parchment paper.

2. Place the broccoli and cauliflower florets on the baking tray, then drizzle with olive oil, sprinkle with pepper and salt, and squeeze a quarter of the juice of the lemon over them. Toss lightly to coat the florets.

3. Place the baking tray in the oven and cook for about 20 minutes.

4. Take the florets out of the oven and allow to cool. Transfer to a bowl and add olive oil, a quarter of the juice of the lemon, and salt. Toss lightly to coat evenly.

5. In a separate bowl, combine all the sauce ingredients and mix together well.

6. Assemble the tuna bowls. Start by filling them with the roasted veggies, top with one can of tuna (for each bowl), and coat them with the sauce.

White Fish Cakes with Aioli

These fish cakes are perfect as a light meal or as an accompaniment to other dishes. You can use whichever white fish you prefer for this dish. The great thing about white fish is that they contain high amounts of protein, and you can easily serve them with healthy fats to up your fat intake for the day.

Time: 45 minutes

Serving Size: 18 patties (depending on the size)

Ingredients for the fish cakes:

- 1 tsp cumin (ground)
- 1 tsp lemon zest (fresh)
- 2 tbsp parsley (chopped)
- 4 tbsp flax meal
- 4 tbsp ghee
- ½ cup parmesan cheese (grated)
- 2 cups cauliflower (riced, cooked)

- 1 ½ lb cod fillets (boneless and skinless—you can use other white fish, too)

- 1 large spring onion (chopped)

- 1 garlic clove (minced)

- 2 large eggs

- black pepper (freshly ground)

- salt

Ingredients for the aioli dip:

- ½ cup mayonnaise

- 2 garlic cloves (minced)

Directions:

1. Add a tablespoon of ghee to a saucepan, along with the minced garlic. Cook over medium heat until fragrant.

2. Add the cooked cauliflower rice, then season with pepper and salt. Cook for 5 to 7 minutes while stirring continuously until tender and crisp.

3. Transfer the cauliflower to a bowl and set aside.

4. Season the fish fillets with pepper and salt.

5. Add a tablespoon of ghee to the same saucepan and cook the fillets over medium-high heat for about 2 to 3 minutes for each side. You know the fillets are cooked when they're flaky and opaque.

6. Transfer the fish to a bowl and allow to cool for about 5 to 10 minutes.

7. After the fish has cooled, add the cauliflower rice and all the other ingredients to the bowl. Mix well to combine.

8. Take portions of the mixture and shape them into patties. The number of patties you can make from this mixture depends on the size and thickness you are looking for.

9. Add a tablespoon of ghee to a pan on

medium-high heat. Once the pan is hot, lower to medium heat and begin placing the patties in the pan. Cook the patties for about 3 to 5 minutes on each side.

10. Combine the sauce ingredients and mix well. Serve the patties hot with the aioli dipping sauce.

Baked Wild Salmon with Fennel and Asparagus

If you're looking for a simple recipe that requires little prep work, this is the one for you. The coconut aminos marinade of this dish has a unique umami flavor that suits the fish perfectly. Pair this with asparagus and fennel and you have a filling and healthy dish to enjoy in less than an hour.

Time: 40 minutes

Serving Size: 4 servings

Ingredients:

- 1 tsp Himalayan pink salt
- 1 tbsp coconut aminos
- 1 tbsp honey
- 1 tbsp kelp (dried)
- 1 tbsp lemon juice (fresh)
- 1 tbsp olive oil

- ½ cup fennel (sliced thinly)

- 2 cups asparagus

- 1 ⅓ lbs salmon (wild, any variety)

- 2 medium-sized avocados (sliced)

- chili flakes (optional)

- fennel fronds

Directions:

1. In a small bowl, combine coconut aminos, honey, kelp, lemon juice, and salt, then mix well to combine—this serves as the marinade.

2. In a bowl, add salmon and the marinade. Mix well, then allow to marinate for about 30 minutes.

3. While waiting, steam the asparagus then set aside to cool.

4. Preheat your oven to 350°F and line an oven pan with parchment paper.

5. Add fennel to the oven pan and place

the marinated salmon on top.

6. Place the pan in the oven and bake for about 10 minutes.

7. Take the pan out of the oven and transfer the salmon and fennel to plates. Garnish with avocado slices, fennel fronds, chili flakes, and a drizzle of olive oil.

Fried Sardines and Olives

If you're feeling adventurous, you may want to try this quick and simple dish. You can enjoy it as a side dish or even an unconventional snack! Sardines are an excellent type of fish to eat on keto and, paired with olives, this dish will fill you up with a lot of nutrients.

Time: 5 minutes

Serving Size: 1 serving

Ingredients:

- 1 tsp parsley flakes
- 1 tbsp garlic flakes
- 1 tbsp olive oil
- 1 can of sardines (3.5 ounces, in olive oil)
- 5 black olives (sliced roughly)

Directions:

1. Heat up the olive oil in a pan.

2. Add the rest of the ingredients in the pan and fry them together for 5 minutes, stirring continuously.

3. Serve hot.

Pan-Cooked Halibut with a Parmesan Crust

This dish creates a perfect combination. Halibut has a mild flavor and a firm texture, while the parmesan crust perfectly complements its taste and texture. This is another easy recipe where you can use any type of white fish as a replacement for the halibut.

Time: 30 minutes

Serving Size: 6 servings

Ingredients:

- 2 tsp garlic powder
- 1 tbsp bread crumbs
- 1 tbsp parsley (dried)
- 3 tbsp parmesan (grated)
- 1 stick of butter (softened)
- 6 halibut fillets
- black pepper
- kosher salt

Directions:

1. Preheat your oven to 400°F and line a baking sheet with parchment paper.

2. Combine all of the ingredients, except the halibut, and mix well.

3. Use a paper towel to pat the halibut fillets dry, then lay them on the baking sheet.

4. Spread the mixture over each of the fillets, making sure that it covers the whole surface of each fillet.

5. Place the baking sheet in the oven and cook the halibut for about 10 to 12 minutes. Then, turn up the heat to 425°F and continue cooking for about 2 to 3 minutes until golden brown.

Spicy Tuna and Cucumber Rolls

This is another easy meal that you can whip up in a matter of minutes. It's rich in protein and it's packed with flavor, too. If you love spicy food and you're looking for something simple to satisfy your cravings, look no further.

Time: 5 minutes

Serving Size: 1 serving

Ingredients for the rolls:

- 1 tbsp mayonnaise
- 2 tsp garlic powder
- 2 tsp sriracha
- 1 can of tuna (5-ounces)
- 1 avocado (sliced the same width as the cucumber strips)
- 1 medium-sized cucumber
- black pepper
- salt

Ingredients for the sauce:

- 2 tbsp mayonnaise

- 2 tbsp sriracha

Directions:

1. Use a vegetable peeler to create thin cucumber strips.

2. If the tuna has any excess liquid or oil, drain first. Combine the tuna with mayonnaise, garlic powder, sriracha, pepper, and salt, then mix well. The mixture should be moist, not wet.

3. Assemble the rolls. Start by placing a cucumber strip on a flat surface. Spread the tuna mixture along the strip, but leave a 1-inch space at the end.

4. Place the sliced avocado at the end of the strip, then start rolling tightly.

5. Make the sauce by mixing the ingredients together well. Drizzle the sauce over the rolls and serve.

Halibut Ceviche

If you love sushi, poke, and other plates with raw fish, then you'll love this ceviche dish, too. It's an excellent recipe to start with if this is your first time preparing raw fish. And the best part about this recipe is that you can easily customize it according to your own taste.

Time: 10 minutes

Serving Size: 2 servings

Ingredients:

- 2 tsp Brain Octane Oil

- 2 tbsp cilantro (fresh, chopped)

- 2 tbsp pickled radishes (minced finely, optional)

- ½ lb halibut (wild, sushi-grade, cubed)

- 1 green onion (sliced)

- 1 lime (juiced)

- 1 small-sized avocado (cubed)

- black pepper

- salt

Directions:

1. In a bowl, combine the Brain Octane Oil, lime juice, and salt, then whisk to combine.

2. Add the remaining ingredients and toss gently.

3. Divide the mixture into two portions and serve immediately. If you don't use sushi-grade fish, you may place in the refrigerator for a couple of hours, allowing the lime juice to "cook" the fish.

Smoked Salmon Salad with Peppercorns

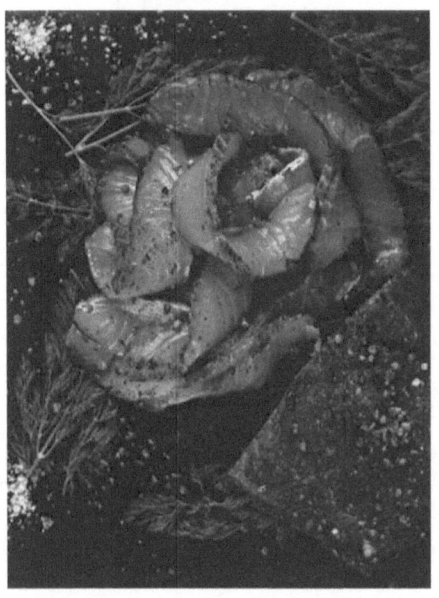

This recipe looks amazing, tastes great, and it's so easy to make. You can enjoy this salad as a light meal, an appetizer, or a side to a heavier meal. However you plan to eat this dish, it's sure to please you.

Time: 5 minutes

Serving Size: 1 serving

Ingredients:

- 1 tsp pink peppercorns (crushed lightly)

- ¼ cup salmon (smoked)

- 1 handful of arugula leaves

- 1 lemon slice

- 4 olives (sliced)

Directions:

1. On a plate, place the olives and arugula leaves.

2. Top the salad with smoked salmon.

3. Lightly sprinkle the salmon with pink peppercorns.

4. Garnish with a lemon slice and serve.

Blackened Tilapia Tacos

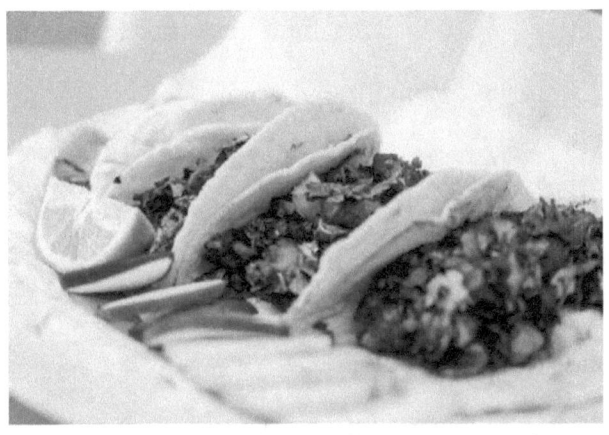

This unique recipe packs a ton of flavors. It's filling, healthy, and it will help you stick with your keto diet. But if you're planning to serve these tacos at a party, it's recommended to make the tortillas in advance as the process may take time. That way, all you have to do is prepare the fillings and start assembling!

Time: 1 hour and 30 minutes

Serving Size: 5 tacos

Ingredients for the taco shells:

- ¼ tsp keto-friendly sweetener (like xanthan gum)

- ½ tsp curry powder

- 2 tsp olive oil

- 2 tbsp psyllium husk (powdered)

- 1 cup filtered water

- 1 cup golden flax meal

- coconut flour

- olive oil

Ingredients for the tilapia:

- 1 tsp chili powder

- 1 tsp paprika

- 5 tilapia fillets

- black pepper

- salt

Ingredients for the slaw:

- 1 tsp apple cider vinegar

- 1 tbsp lime juice

- 1 tbsp olive oil

- ½ cup red cabbage (chopped thinly)

Ingredients for the tacos:

- cilantro (chopped)

- guacamole

- lime slices

- sour cream

Directions:

1. Combine all of the dry taco shell ingredients, then add 2 teaspoons of olive oil and 1 cup of water.

2. Mix well to form a light dough. Set the dough aside, uncovered, for an hour.

3. Divide the dough into 5 blocks. Roll each block over coconut flour to form taco shells. You can also use a tortilla press for this task.

4. Roll out the taco shells as thin as possible then use a round object to cut out the right shape.

5. Heat olive oil in a pan over medium-

high heat and fry the taco shells one by one.

6. In a bowl, combine all of the slaw ingredients. Mix well to combine and set aside.

7. Use paprika, chili powder, pepper, and salt to generously season both sides of the tilapia fillets.

8. Heat olive oil in a pan. Once hot, place the fillets and cook for 3 minutes on each side. Make sure the outside gets blackened.

9. Take the fillets out of the pan and set aside to cool.

10. Assemble the tacos. Start with the tilapia fillets, cabbage slaw, sour cream, and guacamole. Squeeze lime juice over each taco and garnish with fresh cilantro.

Skillet Buttered Cod

This is another quick and simple recipe that comes with all the right flavors—butter, lemon, and herbs. It looks complicated, but you can actually finish the dish in a matter of minutes. It's the perfect meal for lazy days.

Time: 10 minutes

Serving Size: 4 servings

Ingredients for the fish:

- 6 tbsp butter (unsalted)
- 4 cod fillets

Ingredients for the seasoning:

- ¼ tsp garlic powder
- ¼ tsp pepper (ground)
- ½ tsp salt
- ¾ tsp paprika (ground)
- lemon slices
- fresh herbs (parsley or cilantro)

Directions:

1. In a bowl, combine the seasoning ingredients and mix well.

2. Generously season the cod fillets.

3. In a skillet, heat 2 tablespoons of butter on medium-high heat. Add the cod fillets and cook for about 2 minutes.

4. Lower the heat to medium, flip the cod fillets, add the remaining butter, and continue cooking for about 3 to 4 more minutes.

5. Take the skillet off the heat, drizzle with lemon juice, and top with herbs. Serve immediately.

Baked Pesto Sea Bass

This recipe calls for common ingredients—but combining these simple elements creates a stellar dish. Since sea bass is relatively low in fat, the other ingredients add to the fat content of this dish while enhancing the flavor, as well.

Time: 15 minutes

Serving Size: 2 servings

Ingredients:

- 1 tbsp butter, coconut oil, or ghee

- 1 tbsp lemon juice (fresh)

- 4 tbsp pesto

- 2 sea bass fillets

- salt

Directions:

1. Preheat your oven to 400°F and line a baking dish with parchment paper.

2. Place the sea bass fillets on the baking dish, skin side down. Brush the surface with butter, sprinkle salt, and drizzle with lemon juice.

3. Place the baking dish in the oven and cook the sea bass fillets for about 10 minutes.

4. Take the baking dish out of the oven, then top each sea bass fillet with pesto. Spread over the entire surface of each fillet.

5. Place the baking dish back in the oven and continue baking for 3 to 5 minutes more.

6. Take the baking dish out of the oven and allow the sea bass fillets to cool for about 5 minutes before serving.

Grilled Swordfish on Skewers

Virtually anything skewered and grilled is a treat to eat. This time, you will be serving up a unique dish by using swordfish and pesto mayonnaise. The great thing about this recipe is that you can use other kinds of firm fish and seafood to switch it up.

Time: 20 minutes

Serving Size: 4 skewers

Ingredients for the skewers:

- 1 tsp olive oil

- 1 lb swordfish (cubed)

- 16 cherry tomatoes

- black pepper

- salt

Ingredients for the sauce:

- ¼ cup mayonnaise

- ¼ cup pesto

Directions:

1. Divide the cubed swordfish into four portions.

2. Alternately insert cherry tomatoes and swordfish cubes on your skewer.

3. Season with pepper and salt, then drizzle with olive oil.

4. Preheat your grill for about 5 minutes before placing your skewers.

5. Cook for 1 minute on each side of the swordfish cubes. Cooking time will depend on the thickness of your swordfish cubes—for thicker cubes, you may have to cook them for more than 2 minutes. Just make sure to check as you're cooking.

6. To make the sauce, combine the ingredients and mix well. Serve the skewers and sauce together.

Halibut Pescados Asado

For a unique cultural and flavorful dish, you can whip up this fish recipe in your kitchen. As with the other recipes that require white fish, you can replace the halibut with other types of fish as per your preference or product availability. Just wait until you can sink your teeth into this flavor combination!

Time: 10 minutes

Serving Size: 3 servings

Ingredients:

- 1 tsp red pepper flakes

- 2 tbsp cilantro (chopped)

- ¼ cup macadamia oil

- 1 ½ lbs halibut (cut into pieces)

- ½ lemon (juiced)

- ½ lime (juiced)

- 2 scallions (chopped)

- 3 cloves of garlic (minced)

- black pepper

- salt

Directions:

1. In a bowl, combine all of the ingredients except the halibut. Whisk to incorporate well.

2. Place the halibut pieces in a shallow baking dish, then pour over the marinade and toss lightly to coat.

3. Cover the baking dish and place in the refrigerator to marinate for 2 to 3 hours.

4. Preheat your grill and grease the grates using ghee or macadamia oil. Place the marinated fish on the grill.

5. Cook the fish for 5 minutes each side. You know the fish is done when it flakes easily and is opaque. Place the fish on plates and serve hot.

Chapter 4:
Keto-Friendly Seafood Recipes

When it comes to eating fish on keto, there are endless possibilities—and this applies to other types of seafood, as well. Fish and seafood are excellent protein sources and the more dishes you can make using seafood, the more varied and interesting your keto diet can be. Now that you have already learned some simple, easy, and scrumptious fish recipes, it's time to move on to other seafood options. Read on to learn more!

Seared Scallops Topped with Wasabi Mayo

This is a deliciously light option that you can serve as an appetizer, a side dish, or a meal on its own. Gently searing scallops brings out their flavor, especially when you use a lot of butter! Then, topping the scallops off with wasabi mayo makes for a perfect combination.

Time: 20 minutes

Serving Size: 2 servings

Ingredients:

- 1 tsp wasabi paste

- 1 tsp water

- 1 tbsp butter

- 2 tbsp mayonnaise

- 2 slices ginger (pickled, chopped)

- 8 large sea scallops

- black pepper

- chives (chopped)

- salt

Directions:

1. Combine the wasabi paste and mayonnaise and mix well to incorporate.

2. Use a paper towel to pat the scallops dry and season with salt and pepper.

3. In a skillet, heat the butter over medium-high heat. When the butter starts to brown, add the scallops and sear for about 1 ½ minute on each side.

4. Place the scallops on two plates—4 scallops each—and add a dollop of wasabi mayo.

5. Finalize by topping with pickled ginger and fresh chives. Serve immediately.

Lobster-Stuffed Avocado

When most people hear the word "lobster," they immediately think of fine-dining restaurants. But the more you practice cooking seafood, the more you'll realize that lobster can be a part of your regular diet—not just something to indulge in on special occasions. Here's one dish to prove this.

Time: 15 minutes

Serving Size: 4 servings

Ingredients:

- 1 tbsp avocado oil mayonnaise

- 1 tbsp lemon juice (fresh)

- 2 tbsp butter (melted)

- 2 cups lobster meat (chopped, cooled at room temperature)

- 2 California avocados (halved, pitted)

- 1 celery stalk (chopped)

- 1 green onion (chopped)

- black pepper

- chives (fresh, chopped)

- salt

Directions:

1. In a bowl, combine the lobster meat, green onion, and celery.

2. Add the mayonnaise, lemon juice, and butter, then toss lightly to coat evenly. Season with salt and pepper.

3. Use a spoon to scoop out some of the avocado flesh. Just leave about half an inch of flesh.

4. Spoon the lobster mixture into the avocado halves—about half a cup for each.

5. Garnish with chives and serve immediately.

Mexican Shrimp Gazpacho

If you love gazpacho, then you're sure to love this twist to the classic Mexican dish. The tasty seafood mixed with the soup creates a match made in heaven. This keto-friendly dish bursts with vibrant flavors that you'll want to enjoy all year long.

Time: 3 hours and 15 minutes

Serving Size: 4 servings

Ingredients for the soup:

- ½ tsp cumin
- 1 tbsp balsamic vinegar
- ½ cup olive oil
- 5 ½ cups tomatoes (on the vine)
- 1 garlic clove
- 1 jalapeño
- 1 lime (juiced)
- 1 medium-sized cucumber
- 1 medium-sized red onion

- ½ red bell pepper

- sea salt

Ingredients for the shrimp:

- ½ tsp garlic powder

- ½ tsp paprika

- ½ tsp sea salt

- ½ tbsp olive oil

- ½ lb shrimp (peeled, deveined)

Ingredients for the toppings:

- 2 tbsp cucumber (diced)

- 2 tbsp red onion (minced)

- 2 tbsp tomato (diced)

- 1 jalapeño (sliced thinly)

- 1 medium-sized avocado (sliced)

Directions:

1. Roughly chop the soup vegetables then place in a blender. Add the cumin, balsamic vinegar, and lime juice, then blend until you achieve a smooth consistency.

2. Keep the blender running on low, remove the lid, and pour the olive oil slowly until the consistency becomes creamy. Season with sea salt, transfer the soup to a different container, and chill for a minimum of 3 hours.

3. Prepare the shrimp right before serving the gazpacho. In a small bowl, combine all of the shrimp ingredients and toss lightly to coat evenly.

4. Heat a skillet over medium-high heat, add the shrimps, and cook for about 3 to 4 minutes each side.

5. Take the soup out of the refrigerator, spoon into bowls, and top with the shrimp. Finish it off by adding the cucumber, red onion, tomato, jalapeño, and avocado, then serve.

Manhattan Clam Chowder

This hearty, healthy soup is simple to make and is perfectly low-carb, too. Instead of using potatoes, which have a high carb content, you can use celery root instead. Whip up this gourmet chowder to keep yourself warm whenever it's cold.

Time: 30 minutes

Serving Size: 8 servings

Ingredients:

- ½ tsp thyme (dried)
- 2 tbsp tomato paste
- 6 tbsp butter
- ¼ cup parsley (fresh, chopped)
- ½ cup bell pepper (diced)
- ½ cup carrot (chopped)
- ½ cup dry white wine
- ½ cup onion (diced)

- 1 cup clam juice

- 1 ¼ cup celery root (peeled, diced)

- 1 ¾ cup plum tomatoes (whole with juice)

- 2 ½ cup whole baby clams (canned with liquid)

- 4 cups chicken broth (unsalted)

- ⅓ lb bacon (diced)

- 2 bay leaves

- 2 large garlic cloves (roughly chopped)

- black pepper

- salt

Directions:

1. Heat a soup pot over medium heat. Once hot, add a small amount of oil along with the diced bacon. Cook the bacon until crispy, stirring occasionally for about 5 minutes.

2. Turn down the heat to medium-low then add

bell pepper, carrot, onion, celery root, and garlic. Continue stirring to evenly coat the veggies with bacon grease.

3. Add the wine and cover the pot. Allow the veggies to sweat for 2 to 3 minutes.

4. Open the lid, stir, then add in the bay leaves, tomato paste, and thyme.

5. Crush the tomatoes and add them to the pot with the liquid. Also, add the clam juice and chicken broth.

6. Turn up the heat to medium-high and bring the chowder to a boil. Once it starts boiling, return the heat to medium-low and allow the chowder to simmer for about 15 minutes.

7. Add the clams and continue simmering. Also, add the butter and stir until melted.

8. Add salt and a lot of pepper to bring out the soup's savory flavor. Finally, stir the parsley in, then serve hot.

Fried Soft Shell Crab

Who doesn't like fried food? This dish is crunchy, savory, and completely irresistible. Take a break from the usual crab dishes by whipping up a batch of soft shell crabs that are breaded and fried to perfection.

Time: 16 minutes

Serving Size: 2 servings

Ingredients:

- 4 tbsp barbecue sauce

- ½ cup lard

- ½ cup parmesan cheese (powdered)

- 2 eggs (beaten)

- 8 soft shell crabs

Directions:

1. Heat a skillet with lard over medium-high heat.

2. Use a paper towel to pat the crabs dry.

3. Prepare the parmesan and eggs by placing them in separate shallow dishes.

4. Dip one crab into the egg, tap off any excess, and dip into the parmesan cheese. Make sure the crab is coated well and evenly.

5. Drop batches of crabs into the oil and cook for about 2 minutes on each side.

6. Serve the crabs hot with barbecue sauce for dipping.

Poblano Peppers Stuffed with Cajun Shrimp

Peppers are great—you can stuff them with virtually anything, including meat, seafood, cheese, and more. For the final step of cooking, you can either bake or stuff your peppers. This versatile recipe can be changed in different ways depending on your own preference. To give you a better idea of how easy it is to prepare stuffed peppers, here's a simple recipe for you.

Time: 55 minutes

Serving Size: 2 servings

Ingredients:

- 2 tsp olive oil

- 1 tbsp Cajun seasoning mix (or more, if you prefer)

- 1 tbsp hot sauce of your choice

- ½ cup goat cheese

- ½ cup Manchego cheese (shredded)

- 1 cup onion (chopped)

- 1 cup shrimp (peeled, deveined)

- 1 jalapeño (chopped)

- 2 large poblano peppers

- 2 garlic cloves (chopped)

- 12 basil leaves (shredded)

- cilantro (fresh, chopped)

Directions:

1. Place the poblano peppers on a greased baking sheet and broil in the oven. The skin should char and puff up.

2. Take the peppers out of the oven, allow to cool for a bit, then start peeling off the skins.

3. Slice the peppers in half and use a spoon to scoop out the seeds. Place the peppers on a large baking sheet lined with parchment paper.

4. In a bowl, combine the shrimp with olive oil and the Cajun seasoning mix. Toss lightly to coat the shrimps.

5. Heat olive oil in a pan over medium heat. Cook the jalapeño and onion for 5 minutes to soften them up.

6. Add the garlic and continue cooking for another minute. Transfer the cooked veggies to a bowl.

7. Place the shrimp in the same pan and cook for 2 to 3 minutes on each side.

8. Take the shrimp out of the pan, cool for a bit, then chop roughly and add to the cooked vegetables.

9. Add the basil leaves, cheeses, and hot sauce, then mix well.

10. Generously spoon the mixture into the broiled peppers.

11. Place the baking sheet into the oven and bake the peppers for 20 to 30 minutes at 375°F.

12. Top with cilantro and serve hot.

Lobster Cobb Salad

This recipe adds a light and summery twist to the classic Cobb salad. It's an easy dish that is another opportunity to use lobster in a tasty and healthy way. You can either cook the lobster yourself or have it steamed at the seafood store. You can also use shrimp or crab in place of lobster for this recipe.

Time: 20 minutes

Serving Size: 2 servings

Ingredients for the salad:

- ¼ cup avocado (diced)

- ½ cup corn kernels (cooked)

- ½ cup grape tomatoes (quartered)

- 1 ¼ cups lobster meat (cooked, chilled, chopped)

- 2 cups baby greens

- 2 eggs (hard-boiled, sliced)

- 4 strips of bacon (cooked, crumbled)

Ingredients for the dressing:

- 1 tsp dijon mustard

- 4 tsp olive oil

- 2 tbsp red onion (chopped)

- 3 tbsp red wine vinegar

- kosher salt

Directions:

1. Combine all of the dressing ingredients, whisk well, and set aside.

2. Assemble the salad. Start with 1 cup of baby greens, then top with the remaining salad ingredients.

3. Drizzle with the vinaigrette and serve.

Spicy Oyster Stew

These broiled oysters come with a fiery kick! If you're a lover of spicy seafood dishes, this is the perfect recipe for you. It's easy to make, and it only requires five ingredients. It doesn't get any simpler than this—unless you slurp the oysters raw!

Time: 12 minutes

Serving Size: 2 servings

Ingredients:

- 1 tbsp garlic chili paste

- 1 tbsp olive oil

- 12 oysters (shucked)

- 7 basil leaves (fresh)

- salt

Directions:

1. In a bowl, combine olive oil, garlic chili paste, and salt.

2. Add the oysters to the sauce and toss lightly to coat.

3. On a baking dish, lay out all of the basil leaves in a single layer.

4. Pour the oysters and sauce over the basil leaves and spread out evenly.

5. Turn your broiler on high. Place the baking dish on the topmost rack and broil for 2 to 3 minutes.

6. Take the baking dish out of the broiler and serve.

Seared Scallops in Garlic-Lemon Butter

You can't go wrong with seared scallops. Here's another scallop dish that's simple, tangy, silky, and brings out the natural sweet flavors of the juicy shellfish. Enjoy this with a high-fat salad and you'll be feeling full all day.

Time: 15 minutes

Serving Size: 4 servings

Ingredients:

- 1 tbsp chives (fresh, chopped)
- 3 tbsp olive oil
- 4 tbsp butter
- 4 tbsp parsley (fresh, chopped)
- ⅓ cup chicken broth
- 2 cups scallops (fresh, trimmed)
- 1 garlic clove (minced)

- 1 lemon (juiced, zested)

- black pepper

- salt

Directions:

1. Heat the olive oil in a pan over high heat.

2. Once hot, turn the heat down slightly and add the scallops in batches. Cook for about 3 minutes on each side.

3. Remove the scallops from the pan and set aside.

4. In the same pan, add 3 tablespoons of butter and garlic. Cook the garlic until softened. Add chicken broth and continue cooking until slightly thickened.

5. Add 1 tablespoon of butter, lemon zest, lemon juice, and herbs, then mix well.

6. Add the seared scallops to warm through. Serve immediately.

Crab and Bacon-Stuffed Mushrooms

Crab and bacon? What more can you ask for? These two main ingredients are enough to make anyone drool. But once you see (and taste) the final results, you might want to keep cooking this dish over and over again!

Time: 50 minutes

Serving Size: 5 servings

Ingredients:

- 1 tbsp dijon mustard

- ¼ cup sour cream

- ⅓ cup sharp cheddar cheese (shredded)

- ½ cup parmesan cheese (shredded)

- ¾ cup cream cheese (softened)

- 1 ½ cup lump crab meat (fresh)

- 2 cups cremini mushrooms (de-stemmed, cleaned)

- 3 garlic cloves (minced)

- 3 green onions (chopped)

- 6 strips of bacon (cooked, crumbled)

- black pepper

- sea salt

Directions:

1. Preheat your oven to 400°F and use parchment paper to line a baking sheet.

2. Place the mushroom caps on the baking sheet and bake for about 10 minutes.

3. Take the baking sheet out, pour out any excess moisture that has accumulated in the mushroom caps, and set aside.

4. In a bowl, combine the rest of the ingredients except for the parmesan cheese. Mix well to ensure all ingredients are well incorporated.

5. Spoon the crab mixture into each of the mushrooms.

6. Place the baking sheet back in the oven and bake the mushroom caps for 10 more minutes.

7. Take the baking sheet out of the oven, top each mushroom cap with parmesan, and return the baking sheet to the oven.

8. Continue baking the mushroom caps for 5 to 10 more minutes and serve hot.

Mixed Seafood Casserole

This keto-friendly seafood casserole features a creamy base, just enough seasoning, and hints of wine. Adding celery and leeks makes this dish even more flavorful and healthy. But the real stars of this dish are the different kinds of seafood that will surprise you with every bite.

Time: 50 minutes

Serving Size: 6 servings

Ingredients for the seafood:

- ½ tsp Old Bay seasoning
- 1 cup dry white wine
- 1 cup water
- 1 ½ cups cod (cubed)
- 1 ½ cups shrimp (peeled, deveined)
- 2 bay leaves

Ingredients for the veggies:

- 2 tbsp butter
- 2 celery stalks (diced)
- 2 leeks (white part only, cleaned, cut)
- sea salt

Ingredients for the sauce:

- ½ tsp keto-friendly sweetener (like xanthan gum)
- 1 tbsp butter
- 1 cup heavy whipping cream
- sea salt

Ingredients for the topping:

- 2 tsp Old Bay seasoning
- 1 tbsp butter
- 1 tbsp parsley (fresh, chopped)
- ½ cup parmesan cheese (shredded)
- ¼ cup almond flour (super fine)

Directions:

1. Preheat your oven to 400°F.

2. Heat a saucepan over medium-high heat and stir together Old Bay seasoning, dry white wine, water, and bay leaves. Bring to a simmer for about 3 minutes.

3. Turn down the heat to low and continue simmering for 3 more minutes.

4. Add shrimp to the saucepan and allow to simmer until shrimps turn barely opaque. Transfer the shrimp to a bowl and set aside.

5. Add cod to the saucepan and allow to simmer until the cod pieces turn barely opaque. Transfer cod to a separate bowl and set aside.

6. Continue simmering the liquid on medium-high heat to reduce. Once reduced to about 1 cup, remove from the heat, strain, and set aside.

7. In a separate saucepan, heat 2 tablespoons of butter over medium-high heat. Add celery and leeks, then season with sea salt. Cook the vegetables until soft and the edges start turning brown. Remove the saucepan from the heat.

8. In a casserole dish, arrange the vegetables into a single layer. Top with a single layer of seafood . Set aside.

9. In the saucepan used for cooking the vegetables, add 1 tablespoon of butter and the sweetener.

10. Slowly pour the reduced liquid into the saucepan, stirring constantly. Bring the mixture to a boil, reduce heat, and allow to simmer.

11. Once the mixture has thickened, add the whipping cream. Bring to a boil and allow to simmer, stirring constantly. Continue stirring and cooking until you achieve a gravy-like consistency.

12. Once you have the desired consistency, pour the liquid over the seafood and veggies.

13. Combine all of the topping ingredients in a bowl, except for the parsley. Mix well, then sprinkle on top of the casserole.

14. Place the casserole dish in the oven and bake for 20 minutes.

15. Take the casserole dish out of the oven, garnish with parsley, and serve hot.

Shirataki Shrimp Pad Thai

This is a light and flavorful meal that uses shirataki noodles to make it suitable for the keto diet. It's a bright and interesting twist to the classic Thai dish. This pad thai has a fresh and delicate sauce that's delicious whether you eat it right after cooking or have the leftovers cold.

Time: 20 minutes

Serving Size: 3 servings

Ingredients:

- ¼ tsp red pepper (crushed)

- 1 tsp cashew butter

- 1 ½ tbsp Brain Octane Oil

- 2 tbsp coconut aminos

- ¼ cup cilantro

- 1 ¾ cups shirataki noodles (cooked)

- 1 garlic clove (finely minced)

- 1 lime (juiced)

- 2 eggs (beaten)

- 2 green onions (chopped)

- 4 cashews (crushed)

- 18 medium-sized shrimps (wild-caught)

- sea salt

Directions:

1. In a bowl, combine the red pepper, cashew butter, half of the Brain Octane Oil, coconut aminos, garlic, and half of the lime juice.

2. Heat a skillet over medium heat, then add the shrimp, sea salt to taste, and the remaining Brain Octane Oil. Cook the shrimps for about 2 minutes on each side.

3. Move the shrimps to one side of the skillet, then add the eggs. Scramble the eggs for about 1 minute.

4. Add the noodles, the sauce mixture, green onions, and cilantro, then toss everything together to combine.

5. Finish by drizzling the remaining lime juice over the whole skillet and adding more sea salt to taste.

6. Spoon the pad thai onto plates, garnish with crushed cashews, and serve.

Garlic-Butter Baked Lobster Tails

These luscious lobster tails are coated with butter, parmesan cheese, and garlic, then baked to perfection. It's a mouthwatering recipe that you can put together in no time at all. Whip it up for yourself or impress your loved ones with this sophisticated, yet simple concoction.

Time: 15 minutes

Serving Size: 4 servings

Ingredients:

- 1 tsp Italian seasoning mix

- 4 tbsp butter (melted)

- ¼ cup parmesan cheese (grated)

- 1 lemon (juiced)

- 4 lobster tails

- 5 garlic cloves (minced)

- salt

Directions:

1. Preheat your oven to 350°F and line a baking sheet with parchment paper.

2. In a bowl, combine the Italian seasoning mix, butter, parmesan cheese, lemon juice, garlic, and a pinch of salt.

3. Use a sharp pair of scissors to cut off the clear skin from the lobster tails.

4. Brush each of the lobster tails with the garlic butter mixture.

5. Arrange the lobster tails on the baking sheet.

6. Place the baking sheet in the oven and bake the lobster tails for about 15 minutes. You'll know they're done when the lobster meat has become opaque and firm. Serve hot.

Shrimp and Grits with Arugula

Cauliflower is one of the most popular veggies these days because you can cook it in so many different ways and use it in a wide variety of dishes. In this recipe, you will be using cauliflower to make "grits." It's another scrumptious and innovative recipe that has been modified to suit the keto diet.

Time: 30 minutes

Serving Size: 4 servings

Ingredients for the shrimp:

- ½ tsp cayenne pepper

- 2 tsp garlic powder

- 1 tbsp olive oil

- 1 tbsp paprika

- 4 cups shrimps (peeled, deveined)

- black pepper

- salt

Ingredients for the grits:

- 1 tbsp butter (unsalted)

- ½ cup goat cheese (crumbled)

- 1 cup whole milk

- 4 cups cauliflower (riced)

- black pepper

- salt

Ingredients for the arugula:

- 1 tbsp olive oil

- 4 cups baby arugula

- 3 garlic cloves (sliced thinly)

- black pepper

- salt

Directions:

1. Place all of the shrimps in a zip-top bag.

2. In a bowl, combine the cayenne pepper, garlic powder, paprika, pepper, and salt, then mix well.

3. Add this seasoning mixture to the shrimp, seal the bag, and shake to coat the shrimps evenly.

4. Place the bag inside the refrigerator to chill and marinate while you prepare the grits and arugula.

5. Melt butter in a pot over medium heat. Add the riced cauliflower and cook for about 3 minutes to release some moisture.

6. Pour half of the whole milk and bring to a simmer. Stir occasionally while simmering for about 8 minutes.

7. Add the rest of the milk and continue simmering for 10 more minutes until you achieve a creamy and thick consistency.

8. Stir the goat cheese in, add salt and pepper to taste, and keep warm.

9. Heat the olive oil in a skillet over medium heat.

10. Add the garlic and cook for about 1 minute until fragrant.

11. Add the baby arugula and sauté for about 3 minutes until the leaves are wilted.

12. Season with salt and pepper, transfer to a bowl, and set aside.

13. Add more olive oil to the same skillet. Add the seasoned shrimp, then sauté for about 5 minutes.

14. Assemble each plate. Start by spooning the grits onto the plates, top with shrimp and arugula, and serve hot.

Zoodles and Clams with White Sauce

This dish is light, refreshing, and loaded with all the right flavors. It's perfectly simple and it makes for a satisfying dinner. Instead of using high-carb pasta, you'll use zoodles—zucchini noodles.

Time: 20 minutes

Serving Size: 4 servings

Ingredients:

- 1 tsp lemon zest (freshly grated)

- 1 tbsp garlic (minced)

- 2 tbsp lemon juice

- 2 tbsp olive oil

- ¼ cup butter

- ¼ cup parsley (fresh, chopped)

- ½ cup dry white wine

- 4 cups small clams

- 8 cups zoodles

- black pepper

- salt

Directions:

1. Combine the olive oil, butter, salt and pepper in a pan over medium-high heat.

2. Add the garlic and sauté for about 2 minutes until fragrant.

3. Add the lemon juice and wine, then continue cooking until the mixture reduces slightly, about 2 to 3 minutes.

4. Add the small clams and continue cooking for 2 to 3 more minutes or until all of the clams open. If there are any clams that don't open, discard.

5. Remove the pan from the heat and add the zoodles.

6. Toss lightly to coat the zoodles and set aside until the zoodles are soft enough.

7. Stir in the lemon zest and parsley. Garnish with toppings like cheese, bacon, red pepper flakes, and more if desired.

Conclusion:
It's Time to Get Busy in
the Kitchen!

There you have it—all of the basic information you need to start whipping up amazing dishes in the kitchen. Gone are the days when you feel stuck with your diet, bored enough to feel the urge to go back to your previous eating habits. Lack of variety is one issue all new keto dieters have to deal with—but now, this doesn't have to be a concern for you.

One of the most effective, long-term ways to stick with new diets—especially the ketogenic diet, which is fairly restrictive and comes with a number of rules—is to start cooking your own meals. This is probably why you have chosen to purchase this book in the first place. You wanted to bring more variety into your diet by learning how to cook keto-friendly fish and seafood recipes. The great news is that this is exactly what you have learned in this book. Aside from recipes, we even offered informative chapters about fish, seafood, benefits of these healthy foods, and more.

In the first chapter, you learned more about fish—the types to eat, the types to avoid, and why it's a great idea to eat fish while following keto. In the second chapter, you learned the same kind of information about seafood. Learning all of this new information about fish and seafood can help you make better choices when it comes to which types of seafood to include in your diet. Also, learning the benefits of fish and seafood helps you understand why you should be eating more of them as you follow the ketogenic diet.

In chapters three and four, you have learned a number of fish and seafood recipes you can start preparing in your very own kitchen. Whether you're a beginning chef or you've been cooking since even before you started the keto diet, you can easily create these dishes by following the simple steps outlined in these recipes. Now that you're armed with a lot of useful information, it's time to get busy in the kitchen!